Table of Contents

Introduction

The Bulletproof Diet was created in 2014 by Dave Asprey, a technology executive turned biohacking guru. Biohacking, also called do-it-yourself (DIY) biology, refers to the practice of modifying your lifestyle in order to make your body function better and more efficiently.Despite being a successful executive and entrepreneur, Asprey weighed 300 pounds (136.4 kg) by his mid-20s and felt out of touch with his own health.In his New York Times bestseller "The Bulletproof Diet," Asprey tells of his 15-year journey to lose weight and regain his health without adhering to traditional diets. He also claims that you can follow his rubric to achieve the same results.Asprey describes the Bulletproof Diet as an anti-inflammatory program for hunger-free, rapid weight loss and peak performance.Dave Asprey, a former technology executive, created the Bulletproof Diet after spending years fighting to overcome obesity. The anti-inflammatory nature of the diet is meant to promote fast weight loss.

What is the Bulletproof Diet?

So many diets create an all-or-nothing mentality that makes you feel deprived when you follow it and guilty when you "mess up." These diets aren't sustainable and lead to binging, crashing, and just giving up. The Bulletproof Diet isn't like that. It's a realistic approach to eating nutrient-dense fats, protein, and tons of organic vegetables to increase fat burning and send energy levels through the roof.

How It Works

The Bulletproof Diet is a cyclical keto diet, a modified version of the ketogenic diet. It entails eating keto foods — high in fat and low in carbs — for 5–6 days a week, then having 1–2 carb refeed days. On the keto days, you should aim to get 75% of your calories from fat, 20% from protein, and 5% from carbs. This puts you into a state of ketosis, a natural process in which your body burns fat for energy instead of carbs. On the carb refeed days, you're encouraged to eat sweet potato, squash and white rice to increase your daily intake of carbs from approximately 50 grams or less to 300.According to Asprey, the purpose of a carb refeed is to prevent the negative side effects associated with a long-term keto diet, including constipation and kidney stones.

The foundation of the diet is Bulletproof Coffee, or coffee mixed with grass-fed, unsalted butter and medium-chain triglyceride (MCT) oil.Asprey claims that starting your day with this beverage suppresses your hunger while boosting your energy and mental clarity.The Bulletproof Diet also incorporates intermittent fasting, which is the practice of abstaining from food for designated periods.Asprey says that intermittent fasting works in tandem with the Bulletproof Diet because it gives your body steady energy with no crashes or slumps.However, Asprey's definition of intermittent fasting is unclear because he says that you should still consume a cup of Bulletproof Coffee each morning.

Can It Help You Lose Weight?

There are no studies examining the effects of the Bulletproof Diet on weight loss. That said, research indicates that there is no single best diet for weight loss. Low-carb, high-fat diets like the keto diet have been shown to result in quicker weight loss than other diets — but the difference in weight loss seems to disappear over time.The best predictor of weight loss is your ability to follow a reduced-calorie diet for a sustained period.Thus, the Bulletproof Diet's impact on your weight depends on the number of calories you consume and how long you can follow it.Due to their high fat content, keto diets are considered filling and may allow you to eat less and lose weight fairly quickly.That said, the Bulletproof Diet does not restrict calories, suggesting that you can reach a healthy weight through Bulletproof foods alone.Yet weight loss isn't that simple. Your weight is influenced by complex factors, such as genetics, physiology and behavior.Therefore, no matter how "Bulletproof" your diet, you can't always rely solely on your food intake and may have to make a conscious effort to reduce calorie consumption.You must also follow the diet long-term in order for it to

work, which could be challenging for some people.

The Elements of Bulletproofing Your Diet ForAccelerated Fat Loss

In order to effectively follow a diet plan, you have to do your homework and understand it. Knowing why you're doing things not only helps you to stick to the plan, but it also helps you to customize it later on so it will work even better with your own unique biochemistry. So, let's take a close look at the various elements that make up the bullet proofing your diet for shedding fat and reclaiming health.

Ketogenic

Bullet proofing your diet is both low-carb and high-fat, so it's a ketogenic eatingprotocol. This means that you're retraining your body as to what to burn for fuel.The easiest way for our bodies to get energy is to convert carbohydrates to glucose, which is then metabolized for energy. Whatever isn't used is stashedaway in fat deposits for use later as needed. These are your love handles.Your system, however, is fully capable of running off of a higher-octane fuel,ketones. As a matter of fact, newborns are ketogenic, and they stay that way untilwe start feeding them carbohydrates! Ketones are produced from dietary fat,supplying lots of power without the hormonal spikes and cravings that carbs cancause. Just like that high-octane gasoline, they're cleaner burning and give youmore mileage.Why don't we stay as ketogenic as a newborn? Because carb conversion is lesswork for your system and, I'm sorry to say, it can be as lazy as any of us. As long as it has enough carbohydrates, your body will stick with the 'carb-to-glucose-toenergy/fat stash" plan. Controlling, in fact drastically reducing, the amount ofcarbs available will force it to get off the sofa and start doing some work. So, a low carb diet pushes you towards a metabolic state called ketosis, where your system is efficiently using ketones as its major fuel source.However, making ketones requires fat— more fat than we're used to consuming inour modern low-fat world. Our dietary fat consumption is augmented by ourstored body fat in order to provide enough raw material to make all thoseketones. Fat loss, yay! But, if you don't eat enough fat and you've restricted carbs, you have a recipe for disaster. Low-carb dieting requires high-fat eating.Otherwise, your brain interprets low carb and low fat as FAMINE...and it busilystarts storing whatever it can as fat to see it through the coming bad times.This is what derails many diet plans. We'd all love to cut the carbs and live off thespare tire, but it just won't work unless you're actually really starving. Then a hostof other physical problems join the party, such as muscle deterioration including your heart muscle. That's what happens with anorexia, and you don't want to go there.To avoid that, you need to supply your body with usable fuel in the form of fats. A high fat intake is interpreted as PLENTY...and your system doesn't worry aboutstoring fuel to prepare for famine. When it needs a little more, it goes to that pantry it's created around your middle and gets some fat. Basically, you have to eat fat to lose fat, as contradictory as that might seem. For many people, eating enough fat to maintain the state of ketosis is a major hurdle in following a lowcarb diet successfully. Lots of people haven't had full-fat milk in decades, and it can be hard to break the habit of grabbing that low-cal non-fat yogurt! This famine/plenty scenario is what causes the phenomenon known as 'yo-yo dieting'. Your body had reduced fuel available and it has lost weight. When fuel becomes plentiful again, it stores as much as it can to prepare for the next dieting onslaught. The weight comes back (plus some), and so it goes. Your metabolism is on the defensive all the time, torn between famine and plenty, and it can get plenty messed up by that. Enough fat in your diet prevents that yo-yo effect because your brain can't see any hint of famine on the horizon, and your metabolism can function peacefully. You can expect fat loss to average out to about a pound a day on a long-term ketogenic diet. That's loss of body fat, not necessarily weight. There may be times that your overall weight doesn't change although your body contours will. As you lose fat and build muscle, you'll see the difference in the way your clothes fit for instance, but that may not register on the bathroom scale.

Intermittent Fasting

Intermittent fasting simply means going without food for a set interval of time. Unless you're raiding the fridge every two hours all night long, you already do some intermittent fasting...but we usually consider it 'sleeping'. If you skip breakfast, you're actually already fasting for 10 to 16 hours every day. We just don't tend to think of it that way. Although some diets recommend an alternatedays interval, most people find that restricting their food consumption to a specific period of 6-8 hours per day works very well for them. Intermittent fasting by itself can lead to fat loss for a lot of people. There are a lot of current research studies that are focusing on the health benefits of this type of periodic fasting. It appears to help regulate blood sugar, insulin levels, and cholesterol in as little as three weeks. The risk of cancer seems to be lowered by intermittent fasting, as well as our normal rate of cell deterioration, producing an anti-aging effect. One study showed a reduction of up to 45% in the risk of coronary heart disease, and another showed a clear indication that the onset of both diabetes and Alzheimer's could be delayed by regular fasting. These research studies are ongoing, with more positive results being released daily. This type of health benefit is one of the ways you can reclaim your health through by bulletproofing diet, and this type of intermittent fasting is built right into the plan. Breakfast is replaced with high-octane coffee, which keeps you feeling full until lunch and supplies tons of energy, but yet it doesn't metabolically pull you out of the fasting state. You'll have lunch and dinner within a 6 to 8-hour time period in the afternoon and evening, and then return to the fasting state while you sleep.

Anti-Inflammatory

Fighting inflammation is actually where the bulletproof diet began. Asprey discovered that a lot of his health complaints, puffiness, and general malaise stemmed from various sorts of inflammation in his body. He found that various natural as well as artificial toxins found in foods and beverages caused much of this inflammation. Through medical testing, chemical analysis, and selfexperimentation, Asprey bio-hacked eliminating those toxins from his food supply and, in the process, reclaiming a feeling of health and well-being. Coffee makes a good example of how this worked. On some days coffee was energizing and made Asprey feel good; on other days, the same amount of coffee didn't do anything positive at all. Could it be the coffee itself? Upon examining different kinds of coffee, he found that some was higher in mold toxins than others. He discovered through experimenting on himself that the higher the toxins, the worse it made him feel, so he looked for virtually mold-free coffee. Bingo! He got all of the energizing and anti-oxidant effects from coffee without the adverse reactions...and his Upgraded Coffee was born. Extensive research revealed other substances that negatively affect our health in the same way. Just like the otherwise 'benign' mold toxins found in many foods, not just coffee, there are many natural substances that can have the same effect, causing irritation and inflammation that makes us feel terrible. Many chemical and artificial additives in processed food seem to produce the same result, and so do some methods of cooking. That's why eliminating toxins is a large part of the bulletproof diet. This is more than just eating organic, and it sets the bulletproof diet apart from most other eating protocols. Certain foods naturally contain substances, no matter how they're grown or processed, that seem to be dietary irritants and cause inflammation for most people. Generally, removing them from your daily diet will make you feel better. In addition, our bio-individuality means that every person has his/her own personal toxins that will need to be found and eliminated for that person to enjoy optimal health and well-being. This is the tweaking and customization aspect of becoming bulletproof, doing your own bio-hacking and experimenting with these 'suspect' foods.

Timed Eating

The third element of the bulletproof diet involves what's known as timed eating. For most people, coffee is great, even needed, in the morning, but it can cause a lot of problems when drunk too late in the day. That's the basic premise of timed eating, using a food's effect on your body to your advantage. Carbohydrates are well known for providing an energy spike, followed by a crash. They often leave you more tired than you were before, once they burn off. That's the basic problem with a typical carb-laden breakfast—that mid-morning slump. Being bullet proof turns that adverse effect into an asset by moving most of your carbs to your evening meal. You can use the ensuing energy crash to help you to fall asleep more easily at night. The downside of carbs instantly becomes an upside! High-octane coffee is the flipside of the same coin. You're using the caffeine in that coffee to do what it does best, wake you up and sharpen your mental focus. Its effects are positive when experienced in the morning, and they'll be out of your system by evening, so it won't disrupt your sleep. Timing makes all the difference!

Basic Guidelines

Like most diets, the Bulletproof Diet has strict rules that you must follow if you want results. It encourages certain foods while condemning others, recommends specific cooking methods and promotes its own branded products.

What to Eat and Avoid

In the diet plan, Asprey arranges food in a spectrum from "toxic" to

"Bulletproof." You're meant to replace any toxic foods in your diet with Bulletproof ones.

Foods classified as toxic include the following in each food group:

Beverages: Pasteurized milk, soy milk, packaged juice, soda and sports drinks

Veggies: Raw kale and spinach, beets, mushrooms and canned vegetables

Oils and Fats: Chicken fat, vegetable oils, margarines and commercial lard

Nuts and Legumes: Garbanzo beans, dried peas, legumes and peanuts

Dairy: Skim or low-fat milk, non-organic milk or yogurt, cheese and ice-cream

Protein: Factory-farmed meat and high-mercury fish, such as king mackerel and orange roughy

Starch: Oats, buckwheat, quinoa, wheat, corn and potato starch

Fruit: Cantaloupe, raisins, dried fruits, jam, jelly and canned fruit

Spices and Flavorings: Commercial dressings, bouillon and broth

Sweeteners: Sugar, agave, fructose and artificial sweeteners like aspartame

Foods deemed Bulletproof include:

Beverages: Coffee made from Bulletproof Upgraded Coffee beans, green tea and coconut water

Veggies: Cauliflower, asparagus, lettuce, zucchini and cooked broccoli, spinach and brussels sprouts

Oils and Fats: Bulletproof Upgraded MCT Oil, pastured egg yolks, grass-fed butter, fish oil and palm oil

Nuts and Legumes: Coconut, olives, almonds and cashews

Dairy: Organic grass-fed ghee, organic grass-fed butter and colostrum

Protein: Bulletproof Upgraded Whey 2.0, Bulletproof Upgraded Collagen Protein, grass-fed beef and lamb, pastured eggs and salmon

Starch: Sweet potatoes, yam, carrots, white rice, taro and cassava

Fruit: Blackberries, cranberries, raspberries, strawberries and avocado

Spices and Flavorings: Bulletproof Upgraded Chocolate Powder, Bulletproof Upgraded Vanilla, sea salt, cilantro, turmeric, rosemary and thyme

Sweeteners: Xylitol, erythritol, sorbitol, mannitol and stevia

Cooking Methods

Asprey claims that you have to cook foods properly to benefit from their nutrients. He labels the worst cooking methods "kryptonite" and the best "Bulletproof."

Kryptonite cooking methods include:

- Deep-frying or microwaving
- Stir-fried
- Broiled or barbequed
- Bulletproof cooking methods include:

- Raw or uncooked, slightly heated
- Baking at or below 320°F (160°C)
- Pressure cooking

Bulletproof Coffee and Supplements

Bulletproof Coffee is a staple of the diet. This beverage contains Bulletproof-brand coffee beans, MCT oil and grass-fed butter or ghee.The diet recommends drinking Bulletproof Coffee instead of eating breakfast for suppressed hunger, long-lasting energy and mental clarity.Along with the ingredients you need to make Bulletproof Coffee, Asprey sells several other products on his Bulletproof website, ranging from collagen protein to MCT-fortified water.

One-Week Sample Menu

Monday

Breakfast: Bulletproof Coffee with Brain Octane — an MCT oil product — and grass-fed ghee

Lunch: Avocado deviled eggs with salad

Dinner: Bunless burgers with creamy cauliflower

Tuesday

Breakfast: Bulletproof Coffee with Brain Octane and grass-fed ghee

Lunch: Tuna wrap with avocado rolled up in lettuce

Dinner: Hanger steak with herb butter and spinach

Wednesday

Breakfast: Bulletproof Coffee with Brain Octane and grass-fed ghee

Lunch: Creamy broccoli soup with a hard-boiled egg

Dinner: Salmon with cucumbers and brussels sprouts

Thursday

Breakfast: Bulletproof Coffee with Brain Octane and grass-fed ghee

Lunch: Lamb chili

Dinner: Pork chops with asparagus

Friday

Breakfast: Bulletproof Coffee with Brain Octane and grass-fed ghee

Lunch: Baked rosemary chicken thighs with broccoli soup

Dinner: Greek lemon shrimp

Saturday (Refeed Day)

Breakfast: Bulletproof Coffee with Brain Octane and grass-fed ghee

Lunch: Baked sweet potato with almond butter

Dinner: Ginger-cashew butternut soup with carrot fries

Snack: Mixed berries

Sunday

Breakfast: Bulletproof Coffee with Brain Octane and grass-fed ghee

Lunch: Anchovies with zucchini noodles

Dinner: Hamburger soup

Potential Downsides

Keep in mind that the Bulletproof Diet has several drawbacks.Not Rooted in Science The Bulletproof Diet claims to be based on solid scientific evidence, but the findings it relies upon are of poor quality and not applicable to most people.For instance, Asprey cites shoddy data claiming that cereal grains contribute to nutritional deficiencies and that the fiber in brown rice prevents protein digestion.However, cereal grains are often fortified with many important nutrients, and their consumption actually increases — not decreases — your intake of important nutrients.And while it's known that fiber from plant foods like rice decreases the digestibility of some nutrients, the effect is rather small and of no concern as long as you're consuming a well-balanced diet.Asprey also provides oversimplified views of nutrition and human physiology, suggesting that people shouldn't regularly consume fruit since it contains sugar or that all dairy — except ghee — promotes inflammation and disease. In fact, fruit consumption is associated with weight loss, and dairy products have been shown to have anti-inflammatory effects.

Can Be Expensive

The Bulletproof Diet can get expensive. Asprey recommends organic produce and grass-fed meats, stating that they're more nutritious and contain less pesticide residue than their conventional counterparts. However, because these items are much more expensive than their conventional parts, not everyone may be able to afford them. While organically grown produce tends to have lower pesticide residue and may contain greater levels of certain minerals and antioxidants than conventionally grown produce, the differences are probably insignificant to have any real health benefit .The diet also recommends frozen or fresh vegetables over the often more affordable and convenient canned vegetables, despite there being no real health benefit.

Requires Special Products

The Bulletproof line of branded products makes this diet even more expensive. Many of the items in Asprey's food spectrum that rank as Bulletproof are his own branded products. It's highly dubious for any person or company to claim that buying their expensive products will make your diet more successful.

Can Lead to Disordered Eating

Asprey's continual classification of food as "toxic" or "Bulletproof" may lead people to form an unhealthy relationship with food.Consequently, this can lead to an unhealthy obsession with eating so-called healthy foods, termed orthorexia nervosa. One study found that following a strict, all-or-nothing approach to dieting was associated with overeating and weight gain . Another study suggested that strict dieting was associated with the symptoms of an eating disorder and anxiety.

High-Octane Coffee or Tea

You can also use green tea for this beverage, but it's not as effective, especially for weight loss. Start

with the lowest amount of butter
and coconut oil and gradually
increase over the course of a week
or so to avoid 'disaster pants'!

Ingredients:

2 cups low-toxin brewed coffee (or
green tea)

1-2 T grass-fed butter

1-2 T coconut oil

"

Directions:

While the coffee is brewing, put
hot water in a glass blender to preheat it. When you're ready to
make your high-octane coffee,
empty the water. Put all the
Ingredients into the blender. Put
the lid on with a kitchen towel over
it. Holding the lid down with your
hand (and the towel), blend the
beverage until you have a nice
froth on the top. [You can use an
immersion or hand blender but it
won't mix as well.] Pour into your
mug and drink somewhat slowly to

give your body time to process the oils.

Avo-Deviled Eggs

These are great to spice up a meal or to eat as a snack. The avocado adds a lot of good healthy fat and nutrients. Snip a corner off of a small plastic bag and use it to pipe the mixture back into the egg halves.

Ingredients:

8 hard-boiled eggs

1/2 large ripe avocado, mashed

1 tsp. raw apple cider vinegar

1 T organic shallot, minced

½ tsp. celery seed (optional)

Sea salt (to taste)

Organic paprika (to garnish)

Directions:

Slice the eggs in half lengthwise and gently pop the yolks into a bowl. Add the avocado, vinegar, shallot, and celery seed. Mash and mix until well combined. Add salt to taste. Spoon or pipe the mixture into the egg halves and garnish with a sprinkle of paprika.

Baked Burgers

Cooking your burgers in the oven prevents the searing that produces toxic AGEs. The bacon on top adds high-grade fats to fuel your ketone-production. Save a burger or two for lunch tomorrow and freeze any other extras for later.

Ingredients:

2 lbs. ground beef (if not grass-fed, use lean)

2 tsp. ground turmeric

1 T dried rosemary

2 T dried oregano

Sea salt (to taste)

4 slices bacon

Directions:

Preheat oven to 325 degrees F. Make about 8 burgers. Combine the spices and rub them directly onto the burgers. Salt to taste. Put a half-slice of bacon on top of each burger and put them on a flat baking pan with sides. Bake for 15-20 minutes to desired doneness.

Creamy Cauliflower

You can use this recipe to make creamy veggies without using either cream or

cheese. Play around with your favorite mix of herbs!

Ingredients:

½ head of cauliflower, broken into flowerets

3 T grass-fed butter

2 T coconut oil, melted

½ tsp. apple cider vinegar

Your herbs of choice

Sea salt (to taste)

Directions:

Steam the cauliflower until tender.
Put about two-thirds into serving
bowl and

the remaining third into a blender
(or bowl if using a hand blender).
Add the

remaining ingredients and blend until smooth. Pour the blended mixture back

over the cauliflower in the serving bowl.

Burger Salad

The easiest and fastest way to make a very portable lunch is to use your extra

proteins from dinner, supplemented with a basic salad. You may reheat the meat and eat it separately, or simply cut it up or crumble it into your salad. Lettuce is

the only leafy green eaten raw on the bulletproof diet, so get several different

varieties! Also remain aware of how many grams of carb you're adding with your

other veggies. Use MCT oil or very high-quality olive oil for the 'other' oil in the

dressings.

Basic Lunch Salad

½ cups lettuce, mixed varieties

celery, cucumbers, radish, avocado, green onion (suspect) as desired

Basic Salad Dressings

Mix all ingredients in a blender. Refrigerate extra.

Creamy Dressing: ½ avocado or 2 egg yolks, ½ peeled cucumber, 2 T coconut oil, 3 T other oil, 2 T apple Cider vinegar, a pinch of sea salt and stevia,

fresh cilantro or oregano.

Honey Mustard Vinaigrette: ¼ c apple cider vinegar, ¼ c olive oil, 3 T mustard, 2 T raw honey.

Basil Creamy Vinaigrette: ½ avocado, ¼ c olive oil, 2 T other oil, ¼ c apple cider vinegar, fresh basil

Ranch: 1 c mayo (see below), 2 T chopped fresh dill, 1 T apple cider

vinegar, 2 cloves garlic (minced), sea salt (Chill before using.)

Mayo: 1 egg, ¾ c extra light olive oil, ¼ cup other oil, 2-3 tsp. fresh lemon

juice, pinch of salt. If it doesn't firm up, add in an egg yolk.

'Whatever' Stove Top Dinner

This is the quick version of this meal and a 'go-to' for many on the bulletproof diet. It gives you a chance to begin to experiment with the foods.

Ingredients:

1 'green zone' meat

1-2 'green zone' vegetables, chopped

spinach or kale

your choice herbs/spices

Directions:

Put some coconut oil in a pan on medium heat. Lightly brown the meat and then

add the veggies and your leafy greens. Sprinkle in your spices and herbs. Stir,

cover, and let it cook until veggies are tender, usually 10-15 minutes.

Creamy Broccoli Soup

This makes lots, so freeze the extra in serving-sized containers for quick lunches or dinners. Once you're testing dairy, try some shredded raw cheddar on top.

Ingredients:

6-8 cups broccoli florets

3-4 shallots, minced

1 carrot, sliced

4 c bone broth or veggie broth

½ c grass-fed butter

Sea salt to taste

Directions:

Put a dab of butter into a large stockpot and lightly sauté the shallots and carrot. Add the broccoli and cook until it's bright green. Pour in the broth and continue to cook until broccoli is tender. Add the remaining butter and blend (a hand blender works well) until desired consistency. Season with sea salt and serve hot.

Greek Lemon Shrimp

You can use any seafood or even chicken in this recipe for a tasty and attractive

dish that's sure to satisfy.

Ingredients:

1 c chopped leeks

½ c chopped celery

½ c chopped carrot

3 eggs

2 lemons (juiced)

1 T MCT or olive oil

2 c shrimp

Directions:

In a large fry pan, cook the leeks, celery, and carrot over low heat for 5-10 minutes. Add the shrimp (fresh or thawed) and a little water to form a broth. In a bowl, beat the eggs until frothy. Continue beating the eggs as you add in the juice from the lemons and then the oil. Turn off the heat under your fry pan. Remove a little hot broth from the pan and beat it into the lemon/egg mixture. Pour the mixture into the fry pan and stir. Garnish with parsley and serve.

Sausage-Burger Balls

Make lots of these and freeze them for a quick easy lunch. Eat them alone dipped in some salad dressing or toss them on a lunch salad. You can double or triple this recipe without a problem.

Ingredients:

½ lb. spicy sausage or chorizo

½ lb. ground beef

1 egg

oregano or basil (to taste)

Directions:

Preheat oven to 325 degrees F. In a large bowl, mix all the ingredients. Form the mixture into bite-sized mini-meatballs. Cook in a flat baking dish with sides until desired doneness is reached, about 10-15 minutes.

Coconut-Crusted Chicken

You can also use shrimp for this recipe, especially if you can't find pastured chicken. It's delicious and simple to make.

Ingredients:

Shredded unsweetened coconut flakes or powder

Sea salt

Fresh parsley

Dried oregano

1 lb. chicken, cut into strips

2 eggs

Directions:

Preheat oven to 325 degrees F. Mix the coconut, salt, parsley, and oregano in one

bowl. In another bowl, beat the eggs until well blended. Dip the chicken into the

egg and then roll in in the dry mix until coated. Bake until it starts to brown.

Salmon-Cuke Bites

This is a quick, easy, and refreshing lunch. You may substitute zucchini or avocado for the cucumber, or use all three for some variety. You can also put a little salad dressing on them.

Ingredients:

Smoked salmon

Cucumber, cut into ½ inch pieces

Sea salt

Directions:

Cut the salmon into strips, and wrap each strip around a piece of cucumber (or

zucchini or avocado). Season with salt or salad dressing (as desired).

Shepherd's Pie

A low-carb version of an old favorite, this dish is cooked on the stovetop and finished in the oven. Have lots of butter on hand to

make the 'mash' really yummy.
This is definitely a 'comfort food'!

Ingredients:

½ lb. bacon, chopped

2 c shredded carrots

2 c diced celery

2 lbs. ground beef

1 c bone or veggie broth

2 heads cauliflower

1 c butter

Directions:

Cut and steam the cauliflower. Put it in a food processor or blender. Add the

butter and blend until nice and smooth. Set it aside.

Cook the bacon in a large fry pan, and then add the carrots and celery. Continue

cooking for about 5 minutes while you preheat the oven to 350 degrees F. Add the ground beef to the fry pan along with a little salt and about half the broth.

Simmer and stir, adding more broth if it gets dry. Cook until the broth has

evaporated and the beef is cooked through. Spread the beef mixture in the

bottom of a large baking dish with high sides. Spoon the cauliflower on top and

smooth. Bake uncovered for about 30 minutes until top starts to brown.

Cashew-Ginger Butternut Soup

This makes about 2 quarts of soup, so be prepared to save the leftovers. You can either do this in a slow cooker or on the stovetop.

Ingredients:

1 large butternut squash

1 can (14 oz.) coconut milk

1 c bone broth or veggie stock

6 carrots, chopped

1 c raw cashews, chopped

1-inch piece fresh ginger, grated

2 tsp. ground cumin

2 tsp. ground cinnamon

Directions:

Combine all ingredients and cook
for 4-6 hours on low in a slow
cooker or on the

stovetop on low heat, stirring
regularly, for 2-3 hours. Blend to a
smooth

consistency before serving.

Thai Veggie Curry with Rice

This is a great carb re-feed meal that packs a punch. You can switch out the veggies for other 'green zone' ones as you choose.

Ingredients:

1 sweet potato, peeled and diced

1 small butternut squash, peeled, seeded and diced

6 T Thai green curry paste

3 T coconut oil

4 leeks, sliced

2 cans (14 oz. each) coconut milk

2 zucchini, diced

3 limes

Directions:

Heat oven to 350 degrees F. Melt 2 T of the coconut oil and mix with 2 T of the

Thai green curry paste. Toss the sweet potato and squash in this mixture, and

then put it all in a roasting pan. Season with salt and roast for about 30 minutes.

To begin the sauce, melt the remaining 1 T of coconut oil in a fry pan. Cook the

leeks until softened and golden. Stir in the remaining 4 T of the curry paste and

cook for a few minutes. Add the coconut milk and a splash of water and simmer.

Add the roasted vegetables along with the zucchini. Simmer for 10-15 minutes.

Stir in the juice from the limes and serve over rice.

Thoroughly rinse white rice before cooking to be bulletproof. Rinse and rinse

until the water's clear. Then cook as usual.

Sweet Potato Ginger Brownies

Using baked sweet potato and coconut flour instead of wheat flour, these brownies are a great example of bulletproof baking.

Ingredients:

2 c cooked mashed sweet potato (purple ones if you can get them)

3 eggs

¼ c butter

¼ c raw honey

3 T coconut flour

3 T dark cocoa powder

2 tsp. ground cinnamon

½ tsp. ground ginger

¼ tsp. vanilla powder

¼ tsp. baking powder

pinch sea salt

½ c chopped Lindt 90% dark chocolate bar

Directions:

Preheat oven to 350 degrees F. Mix the mashed sweet potato with the eggs,

butter, honey, and vanilla. Combine well. Add in the coconut flour, cocoa powder,

spices, baking powder, and salt. Again mix well. Stir in the chocolate pieces.

Spread the batter in a buttered 8x8 pan. Bake 35-45 minutes until a toothpick

comes out fairly clean. Cool before cutting.

'Whatever' Crock-Pot Dinner

This is the long version of this meal and a 'go-to' for many on busy weekends. Your meal can cook while you're out doing things.

Ingredients:

1 'green zone' meat

1-2 'green zone' vegetables, chopped

spinach or kale

your choice herbs/spices

Directions:

Put some coconut oil in a pan on medium heat. Lightly brown the meat and then add the veggies and your leafy greens. Sprinkle in your spices and herbs. Stir,

cover, and cook on low for 6-8 hours.

Bacon-Wrapped Cube Steak

The butter gives added richness to the cube steak, and the bacon wrap is divine. Serve with mashed cauliflower or a cauli-sweet potato mash.

Ingredients:

1 lb. cube steak

sliced bacon

butter

Directions:

Fold the cube steak in half with a good-sized chunk of butter in the middle. Wrap

with bacon. Cook in a fry pan over medium heat until desired doneness, flipping

from time to time.

Poached Salmon with Lemon-Zested Rice

Simple poached salmon is always a hit, and it gives you great leftovers for salads as well. White wine is a suspect beverage, but you won't be drinking it here and the alcohol cooks off. Substitute water if you'd like to completely avoid wine. The only sin with salmon is to overcook!

Ingredients:

1 to 1 ½ pounds salmon fillets, pin bones removed

sea salt

½ c dry white wine

½ c water

1 shallot, peeled and sliced

several sprigs of fresh dill

a sprig of fresh parsley

Directions:

Put all ingredients except the salmon in a large pan. Bring to a simmer over

medium heat. Season the salmon fillets with a little salt. Place them skin-side

down in the simmering liquid in the pan. Cover and cook about 8 minutes,

depending on the thickness of the fillets.

Serve with white rice that you've spritzed with some lemon juice and stirred a

little grated lemon zest into.

Conclusion

The Bulletproof Diet combines a cyclical ketogenic diet with intermittent fasting. It claims to help you lose up to a pound (0.45 kg) per day while boosting energy and focus. Yet, evidence is lacking. It may be beneficial for appetite control, but some may find it hard to follow. Keep in mind that the diet promotes inaccurate health claims and mandates the purchasing of branded products. Overall, you may be better off following proven dietary tips that won't be as expensive and will promote a healthy relationship with food.